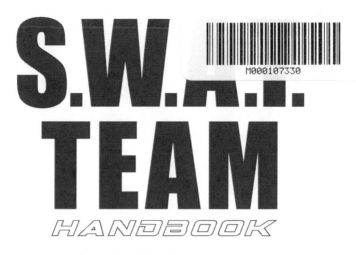

S.W.A.T. TEAM HANDBOOK

Jake DaBell, DDS MSD

S.W.A.T. Team Handbook

Published by Provenir Publishing, LLC, P. O. Box 211, Greenacres, WA 99016-0211

Production Credits

Editor: Amy Hanson

Art Director and Illustration: Micah Harman

Cover Design: Micah Harman

Printing History: January 2014, First Edition.

www.provenirpublishing.com

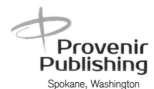

Provenir Publishing
Spokane, Washington

S.W.A.T. TEAM PLEDGE

I PROMISE TO PROTECT AND CARE FOR MY TEETH BY PRACTICING GOOD ORAL HABITS AND AVOIDING HARMFUL ONES AND BY SEEING MY DENTIST AND ORTHODONTIST REGULARLY.

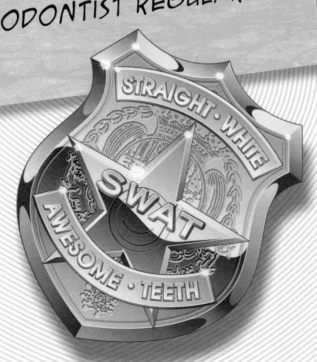

CONTENTS

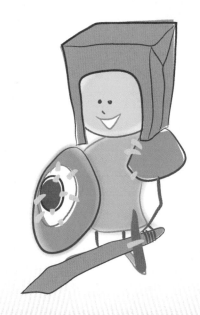

PROTECT YOUR SMILE

The key to an awesome smile is taking good care of your teeth. Your teeth need your help in order to be healthy and to stay looking great. There are many things that your teeth depend on you to do to keep them safe.

BRUSH YOUR TEETH

Your mouth is full of bacteria – little critters that sit on your teeth, your tongue, your cheeks, EVERYWHERE! Some of these tiny creatures take the sugar that you eat and turn it in to acid that breaks

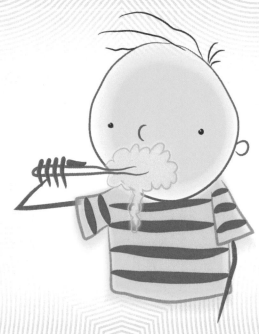

down your teeth and causes white scars on your teeth and cavities. Brushing your teeth cleans the bacteria and the sugar off the teeth and helps prevent white spots and cavities. You should use a soft bristled toothbrush and a small pea size amount of toothpaste with fluoride. Ideally, you should brush after every meal, but at the very least you should brush 2 times per day – in the morning and before you go to bed at night. You should brush for at least 2 minutes each time you brush, so use a timer. When you brush, point the bristles of your toothbrush towards and gums and clean each tooth with a circular brushing motion. Make sure to actually brush your gums – be gentle but thorough. Brush each surface of each tooth – the front, the back, the biting surface and in between the teeth.

- Use a soft bristle toothbrush and fluoride toothpaste.
- Brush at least twice a day for at least two minutes.
- Brush each surface of each tooth, especially by your gums.

FLOSS YOUR TEETH

Flossing your teeth cleans in between your teeth where the tooth brush can't reach. Every place where two teeth contact each other needs to be flossed one time every day. When you floss, pull the floss between two teeth and clean the side of each tooth by wrapping the floss around the side of each tooth, in a C-shape, and moving it up and down, first one tooth and then the other. Flossing is important to get those hard to reach places where bacteria love to hide. It's also important to floss below the gum-line to keep your gums healthy and happy.

- Floss every place where two teeth contact each other one time every day.
- Clean the side of each tooth by wrapping the floss around the side of each tooth, in a C-shape, and moving it up and down.

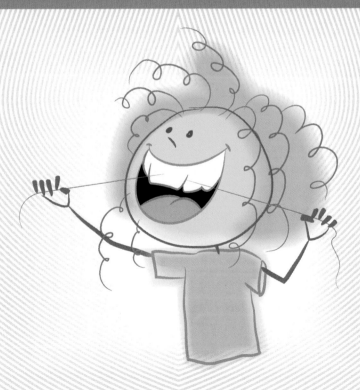

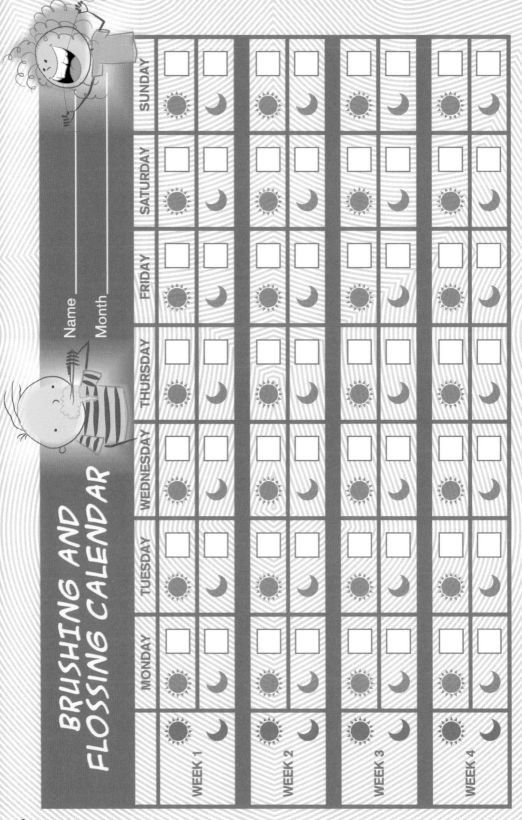

BRUSHING AND FLOSSING CALENDAR

Name

Month

	MONDAY	TUESDAY	WEDNESDAY	THURSDAY	FRIDAY	SATURDAY	SUNDAY
WEEK 1							
WEEK 2							
WEEK 3							
WEEK 4							

8

TOOTH FRIENDLY DIET

The things you eat and drink can affect your teeth. It's important to have a tooth friendly diet to help your teeth stay healthy and strong. Some foods and drinks that are good for your teeth include water, dairy products like milk and cheese, vegetables, especially those high in fiber, and sugar-free gum.

Sugar helps bacteria stick to your teeth. The bacteria turn the sugar into acid which breaks down your teeth and gives you white spots and cavities. A diet low in sugary foods and drinks is important to keep your teeth healthy. If you want to have a sugary treat or a sugary drink, just keep it to meal times and brush your teeth afterwards. Avoid snacking on sugary things or drinking sugary drinks between meals.

Good for your teeth	Bad for your teeth
Water	Soft drinks
Milk, cheese & yogurt	Candy
Vegetables	Citrus fruit
Sugar-free gum	Sugary baked goods

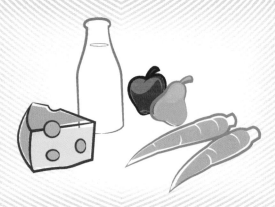

ACIDIC DRINKS

Many of the drinks we drink every day are acidic and can cause damage to your teeth. Many drinks also have large amounts of sugar which can cause scarring on your teeth and lead to cavities. Energy drinks and sports drinks are particularly damaging to your teeth.

This list shows how acidic some popular drinks are and how much sugar they have. The lower the pH, the more acidic the drink is. In drinks with a pH lower than 5.5, the liquid is working to dissolve the enamel on your teeth.

Drink	Acid (pH)	Sugar (tsp. in 12 oz.)
Battery acid (reference)	1.0	
Stomach acid (reference)	2.0	
Lemon juice	2.0-2.6	
Pepsi	2.49	9.8
Country Time Lemonade	2.5	5.4
Coke Classic	2.53	9.3
Capri Sun	2.6	5.5
Powerade	2.75	3.5
Hawaiian Fruit Punch	2.85	9.5
Dr. Pepper	2.92	9.5
Gatorade	2.95	5.5
Fresca	3.2	0
Mountain Dew	3.22	11
Diet Coke	3.39	0
Sprite	3.42	9
A&W Root Beer	4.3	10.7
Coffee	5.51	
Milk	6.8	
Water	7.0	

If you do drink some acidic drinks, here are some tips to minimize the damage done to your teeth. Some of these tips are helpful if you're unable to brush your teeth after eating as well.

- Swish your mouth out with water after drinking these beverages to decrease the acid's contact with your teeth.
- Drink water after consuming an acidic beverage.
- Chew sugar-free gum to increase saliva production (saliva is your mouth's natural rinse).
- Drink sugary or acidic beverages with meals instead of alone.
- Use a straw to help decrease contact with your teeth.
- Brush and floss your teeth twice a day with a fluoride toothpaste.

AVOID TRAUMA

Many problems can result from trauma to the teeth or jaws. One of the best ways to avoid trauma is by wearing a mouth guard if you are participating in a contact sport (football, martial arts, soccer, basketball, rugby, lacrosse, etc). Mouth guards protect your teeth and jaws and are an important part of your equipment.

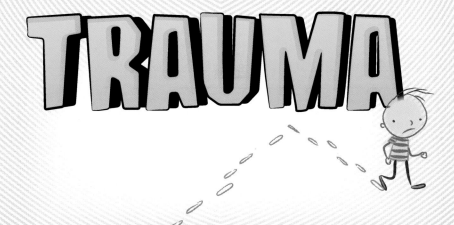

It's also important to know what to do if you have trauma to your teeth. Here are some rules to follow if you ever get hit in the face and break or move a tooth or have a tooth loosened or knocked out.

If the tooth is mobile but still in the correct position:

- Stick to soft foods for the next several days to avoid further trauma to the tooth and to allow it to heal.
- Call your dentist and have the tooth checked to rule out bigger problems.

If the tooth has been moved by the trauma:

- Call your dentist immediately. The tooth will need to be repositioned and examined to determine the best treatment. Your dentist will also want to assess the health of the tooth and check the tooth and bone for fractures.
- Stick to soft foods for the next couple of weeks to allow the tooth and supporting bone to heal.
- The tooth may need to be splinted to heal properly.

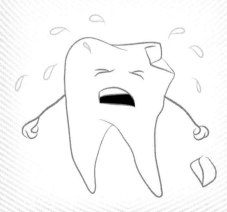

If the tooth has been chipped or broken:

- Your dentist will need to determine the extent of the chip or break and will decide on the right treatment based on where the chip or break is.

If a tooth has been knocked out:

- Keep calm.
- Make sure it is a permanent tooth – baby teeth should not be put back in.
- Find the tooth and pick it up by the crown (the white part). Avoid touching the root.
- If the tooth is dirty, wash it briefly (10 seconds) under cold running water and reposition it. Replant the tooth! Bite on a handkerchief or paper towel to hold it in position.
- If this is not possible, place the tooth in a suitable liquid, like a glass of milk or a special storage liquid for knocked out teeth (such as Hank's Balanced Salt Solution or saline). The tooth can also be transported in the mouth, keeping it between the molars and the inside of the cheek. If the child is very young, he/she could swallow the tooth – therefore it is advisable to get the child to spit in a container and place the tooth in it. Avoid storage in water!
- Seek emergency dental treatment immediately.

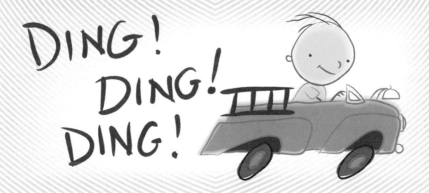

DING!
DING!
DING!

AVOID HARMFUL HABITS

THUMB SUCKING

Children who still suck their fingers or thumbs after their permanent teeth start coming in—usually around the age of 5 or 6—could be causing permanent changes that affect tooth and jaw structure.

BRUSHING TOO HARD

Brushing your teeth regularly is part of good oral hygiene, but brushing your teeth too hard can wear down enamel, irritate your gums, make your teeth sensitive to cold, and even cause cavities. To avoid these problems, use a soft bristled toothbrush.

CHEWING ON ICE

Ice cubes may seem harmless, but chewing on ice can lead to problems. The cold temperature and the hardness of ice cubes can cause serious damage to your teeth.

USING YOUR TEETH AS A TOOL

Many people use their teeth to break off a tag on clothing, rip open a package of potato chips, or even unscrew bottle tops. Using your teeth as a tool is a threat to dental health and can damage dental work or cause your teeth to crack.

NAIL BITING

Biting your nails doesn't just harm the appearance of your hands—it can also damage your teeth. Regularly biting your nails can cause your teeth to move out of place. In addition, nail biting could potentially cause teeth to break or tooth enamel to splinter.

HABIT CALENDAR

The bad habit I'm going to break is: _____

	MONDAY	TUESDAY	WEDNESDAY	THURSDAY	FRIDAY	SATURDAY	SUNDAY
WEEK 1	☀ ☐ ☾ ☐	☀ ☐ ☾ ☐	☀ ☐ ☾ ☐	☀ ☐ ☾ ☐	☀ ☐ ☾ ☐	☀ ☐ ☾ ☐	☀ ☐ ☾ ☐
WEEK 2	☀ ☐ ☾ ☐	☀ ☐ ☾ ☐	☀ ☐ ☾ ☐	☀ ☐ ☾ ☐	☀ ☐ ☾ ☐	☀ ☐ ☾ ☐	☀ ☐ ☾ ☐
WEEK 3	☀ ☐ ☾ ☐	☀ ☐ ☾ ☐	☀ ☐ ☾ ☐	☀ ☐ ☾ ☐	☀ ☐ ☾ ☐	☀ ☐ ☾ ☐	☀ ☐ ☾ ☐
WEEK 4	☀ ☐ ☾ ☐	☀ ☐ ☾ ☐	☀ ☐ ☾ ☐	☀ ☐ ☾ ☐	☀ ☐ ☾ ☐	☀ ☐ ☾ ☐	☀ ☐ ☾ ☐

15

VISIT YOUR DENTIST

One important way to protect your smile and keep your teeth healthy is by visiting your dentist every 6 months for check-ups and cleanings and by getting necessary dental work done when it is recommended. Your dentist is your partner, helping you to keep your teeth shiny and strong. There are lots of things your dentist can do to help you keep your teeth cavity free for a lifetime. Some of these important things are sealants, fluoride treatments and cleanings. So, visit your dentist and be a good patient. It's part of your job as a member of the S.W.A.T. Team!

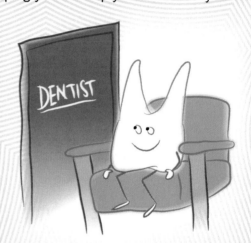

VISIT YOUR ORTHODONTIST

As your teeth, smile and bite develop and grow, sometimes they need some help to develop and grow properly. That's where your orthodontist comes in. Many problems are best corrected early, even when only a few grown up teeth have come in. Other problems are best corrected when all the baby teeth have fallen out and all the permanent teeth have come in. It's your orthodontist's job to know when the best time to correct these problems is and how to correct them. That's why your observation and orthodontic guidance appointments are so important – to do the right treatment at the right time to make your smile and bite the best they can be. After all, that's what the S.W.A.T. Team is all about!

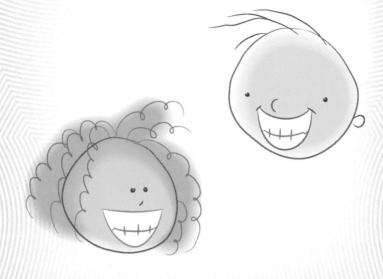

YOUR GROWING SMILE

TYPES OF TEETH

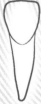 Incisor – Includes central and lateral incisors

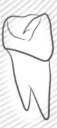 Premolar – Also called a bicuspid

 Canine – Also called a cuspid

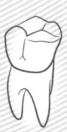 Molar

PRIMARY TEETH
(ALSO CALLED DECIDUOUS TEETH OR BABY TEETH)

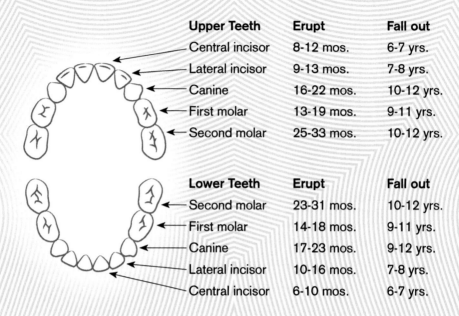

Upper Teeth	Erupt	Fall out
Central incisor	8-12 mos.	6-7 yrs.
Lateral incisor	9-13 mos.	7-8 yrs.
Canine	16-22 mos.	10-12 yrs.
First molar	13-19 mos.	9-11 yrs.
Second molar	25-33 mos.	10-12 yrs.

Lower Teeth	Erupt	Fall out
Second molar	23-31 mos.	10-12 yrs.
First molar	14-18 mos.	9-11 yrs.
Canine	17-23 mos.	9-12 yrs.
Lateral incisor	10-16 mos.	7-8 yrs.
Central incisor	6-10 mos.	6-7 yrs.

WHEN I LOST MY BABY TEETH

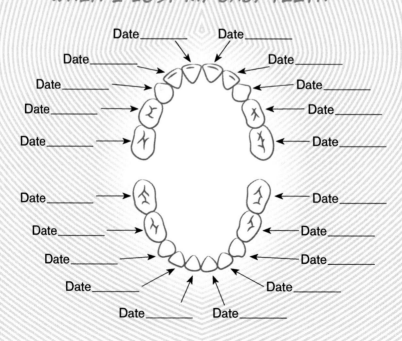

Date_____ Date_____
Date_____ Date_____
Date_____ Date_____
Date_____ Date_____
Date_____ Date_____

Date_____ Date_____
Date_____ Date_____
Date_____ Date_____
Date_____ Date_____

PERMANENT TEETH
(ALSO CALLED SECONDARY TEETH)

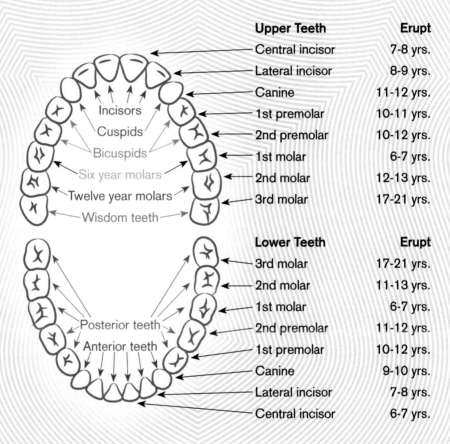

Upper Teeth	Erupt
Central incisor	7-8 yrs.
Lateral incisor	8-9 yrs.
Canine	11-12 yrs.
1st premolar	10-11 yrs.
2nd premolar	10-12 yrs.
1st molar	6-7 yrs.
2nd molar	12-13 yrs.
3rd molar	17-21 yrs.

Lower Teeth	Erupt
3rd molar	17-21 yrs.
2nd molar	11-13 yrs.
1st molar	6-7 yrs.
2nd premolar	11-12 yrs.
1st premolar	10-12 yrs.
Canine	9-10 yrs.
Lateral incisor	7-8 yrs.
Central incisor	6-7 yrs.

Incisors
Cuspids
Bicuspids
Six year molars
Twelve year molars
Wisdom teeth

Posterior teeth
Anterior teeth

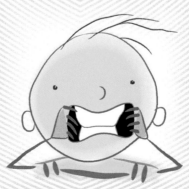

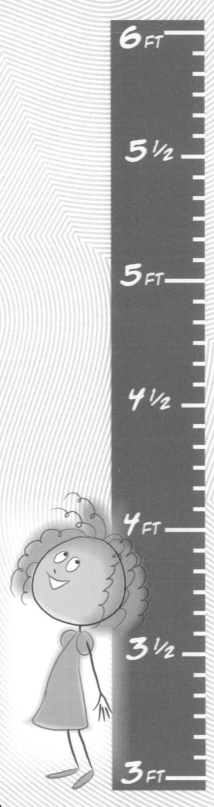

6 FT

5½

5 FT

4½

4 FT

3½

3 FT

GROWTH CHART

Mark your height on the ruler and record the date and height in the space below.

Date_____ Height_____

Date_____ Height_____

Date_____ Height_____

Date_____ Height_____

Date_____ Height_____

Date_____ Height_____

Date_____ Height_____

Date_____ Height_____

Date_____ Height_____

Date_____ Height_____

Date_____ Height_____

Date_____ Height_____

Date_____ Height_____

Dear Tooth Fairy,

How I Lost My Tooth: _____

_____

_____

_____

_____

_____

_____

_____

_____

_____

_____

_____

_____

_____

_____

_____

By _____ Date _____

Dear Tooth Fairy,

How I Lost My Tooth: _____

_____

_____

_____

_____

_____

_____

_____

_____

_____

_____

_____

_____

_____

_____

_____

By _____ Date _____

ORTHODONTIC PROBLEMS TO WATCH FOR

Orthodontic problems are problems of the alignment or the bite of the teeth. Many of these problems can get worse or be more difficult to correct if not taken care of early. This is why it is recommended that children see an orthodontist for the first time at age 7, when the first permanent molars and most of the permanent incisors have grown in. Many orthodontic problems can be seen at this age and can be more easily or more effectively treated at this time. While some problems benefit from early treatment, other problems are best corrected when all the permanent teeth have grown in.

Here are some of the orthodontic problems that can benefit from early treatment. The BEFORE pictures illustrate the orthodontic problem and the AFTER pictures show the teeth after the problem was corrected.

Posterior cross-bite – The top teeth should fit around the bottom teeth when biting like the lid on a box fits around a box. When the top back teeth bite to the inside of the bottom back teeth, it's called a posterior cross-bite.

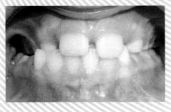
BEFORE

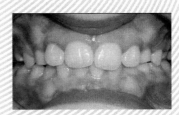
AFTER

Anterior cross-bite – The top front teeth should be in front of the bottom front teeth when biting. When one or more top front teeth bite behind the bottom front teeth, it's called an anterior cross-bite.

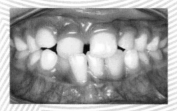

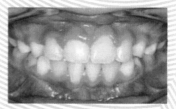

BEFORE   **AFTER**

Underbite – When all the top front teeth bite behind the bottom front teeth, it's called an underbite.

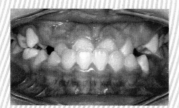

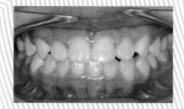

BEFORE   **AFTER**

Protrusive or "buck" teeth – The top front teeth should bite in front of the bottom front teeth, but they should not stick out excessively in front of the bottom front teeth. When the top front teeth do stick out excessively, they are protrusive. They are also often called "buck" teeth.

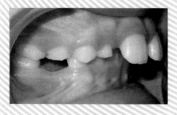

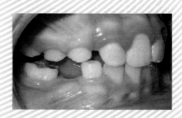

BEFORE   **AFTER**

26

Deep bite – The top and bottom front teeth should overlap when biting together, but the top front teeth should overlap less than half of the bottom front teeth. When the top front teeth overlap most or all of the bottom front teeth, it's called a deep bite.

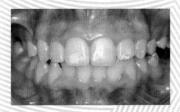

BEFORE

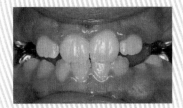

AFTER

Open bite – When the top front teeth don't overlap the bottom front teeth at all, it's called an open bite.

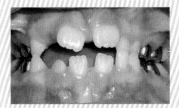

BEFORE

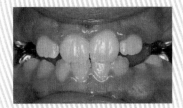

AFTER

Severe crowding – Crowding of the teeth that causes extreme mis-alignment of the teeth or prevents some the permanent teeth from growing in is severe crowding.

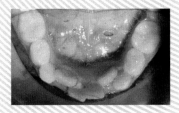

BEFORE

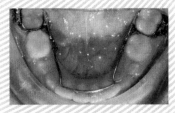

AFTER

Impacted permanent teeth – When permanent teeth don't grow in when they should, sometimes they are impacted and require treatment in order to come into the proper position.

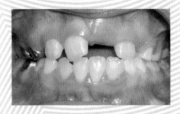

BEFORE

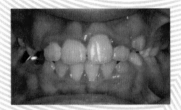

AFTER

Early loss of primary teeth – Baby teeth hold the space for permanent teeth to grow in. When a baby tooth is lost early, some of the space for the permanent tooth may be lost, leading to crowding of the permanent teeth.

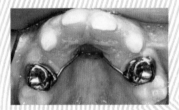

BEFORE

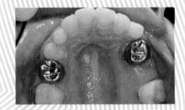

AFTER

Midline diastema – A space between the two top front teeth is called a midline diastema. When this space is large it can be a sign of other problems and may benefit from being closed early.

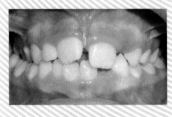

BEFORE

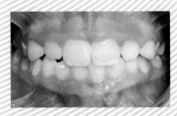

AFTER

These are the types of problems your orthodontist will be watching for at each of your orthodontic growth and guidance appointments. Finding and correcting orthodontic problems at the right time gives you the best chance of growing up with straight, white, awesome teeth.

S.W.A.T. TEAM TRAINING

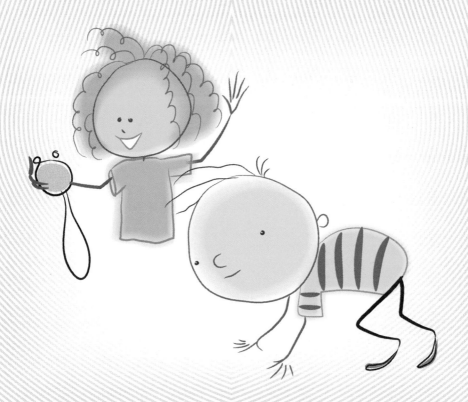

DENTIST VISITS

RECEIVE ONE STAMP FOR EACH APPOINTMENT YOU GO TO WITH YOUR DEN-
TIST FOR A DENTAL CLEANING AND EXAM. ONCE YOU RECEIVE FOUR STAMPS ON
YOUR DENTIST VISIT PAGE AND YOUR ORTHODONTIST VISIT PAGE, YOU WILL BE
AWARDED THE RANK OF S.W.A.T. TEAM CAPTAIN.

ORTHODONTIST VISITS

RECEIVE ONE STAMP FOR EACH APPOINTMENT YOU GO TO WITH YOUR OR-
THODONTIST FOR ORTHODONTIC GROWTH AND GUIDANCE. ONCE YOU RECEIVE
FOUR STAMPS ON YOUR ORTHODONTIST VISIT PAGE AND YOUR DENTIST VISIT
PAGE, YOU WILL BE AWARDED THE RANK OF S.W.AT. TEAM CAPTAIN.

TOOTH TRUTHS QUIZ

1. Who do you see to straighten your teeth?
   - a. the dentist
   - b. the orthodontist
   - c. the hygienist
   - d. none of the above

2. How many permanent teeth do most people have, including wisdom teeth?
   - a. 26
   - b. 32
   - c. 21
   - d. 35

3. How long should you brush your teeth each time?
   - a. 1 minute
   - b. 2-3 minutes
   - c. 30 seconds
   - d. 5 minutes

4. How often should you get your teeth professionally cleaned?
   - a. every 7 months
   - b. every 5 years
   - c. every 6 months
   - d. every 2 years

5. What are the benefits of braces?
- a. straightened teeth
- b. better chewing
- c. better smile
- d. all of the above

6. Which is the best way to keep your teeth healthy?
- a. brush twice a day, floss and visit the dentist regularly
- b. chew gum
- c. use soap and water to brush your teeth
- d. brush your teeth every other day

7. What sticky substance is important to brush off your teeth so you don't get cavities?
- a. toothpaste
- b. gum
- c. plaque
- d. mouthwash

8. _____ means "bad bite" and is used to describe teeth that are crooked, crowded or not lined up properly.
- a. braces
- b. malocclusion
- c. orthodontics
- d. dentistry

Answers on page 41

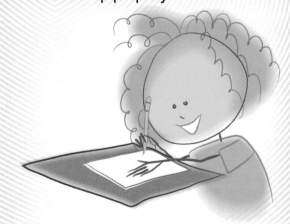

THE TOOTH OF THE MATTER QUIZ .

1. What practice did the Chinese use in 2700 B.C.E. to treat pain associated with tooth decay?
    a. orthodontics
    b. acupuncture
    c. drilling
    d. meditation

2. In 1728, Pierre Fauchard constructed the first "braces" out of a flat strip of metal connected to teeth by _____.
    a. rubber
    b. wire
    c. thread
    d. gum

3. What modern device did New Orleans dentist Levi Spear Parmly invent?
    a. dental floss
    b. dental chair
    c. toothpick
    d. toothbrush

4. What famous "midnight rider" constructed dentures from ivory and gold?
    a. Samuel Adams
    b. Nathan Hale
    c. Paul Revere
    d. Benjamin Franklin

5. If you needed a tooth extracted during the Middle Ages, you would likely visit a _____.
   a. printer
   b. silversmith
   c. weaver
   d. barber

6. What 18th century beauty product caused tooth loss?
   a. lipstick
   b. rouge
   c. nail polish
   d. shampoo

7. What ingredient did ancient Romans apply to their teeth that made them appear shiny but caused decay?
   a. chalk
   b. olive oil
   c. tooth powder
   d. candle wax

8. What U.S. president was nearly toothless, but was meticulous about the teeth of his six white horses that pulled his coach?
   a. George Washington
   b. Abraham Lincoln
   c. Thomas Jefferson
   d. James Madison

9. Which of the following marked a bizarre attempt to treat oral disease during ancient times?

    a. Egyptians would place a live mouse on the gums of a suffering patient because mice had good teeth.

    b. Romans believed that tying a frog to a jaw would make teeth stronger.

    c. Egyptians would apply mixtures made from substances like olive oil, dates, onions, beans, and green lead to teeth.

    d. All of the above

10. Which early dentists invented false teeth almost 3000 years ago?

    a. Sumerians

    b. Etruscans

    c. Persians

    d. Spartans

Answers on page 41

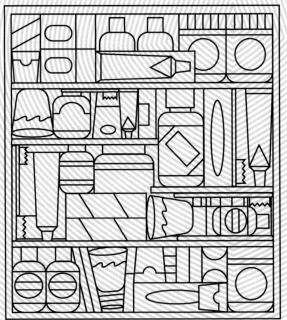

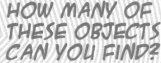

HOW MANY OF THESE OBJECTS CAN YOU FIND?

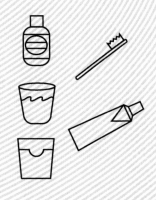

Answers on page 42

FIND ALL OF THE TEETH-RELATED WORDS!

(look in every direction)

```
B R A C K E T B A S H J C I B J
R B P O P N W L O V U O R B A O
A V P L R M I T D F I C C E B C
C T L G I K U R E T A I N E R N
E M I C N O S M I L E S K O U G
S O A P T S V A M T L R D E S U
I N N E A H A M P O I B S C H U
K S C C M G C I R V U A D O A Z
O R E H O G U N E I Z T E J T A
E O R F O L P M S P F D N C R U
Q E W R C O B T S A L A T H K N
A G O E J P A A I P O O I R A D
M H H T E C N H O A I D S A L E
T O R T H O D O N T I S T D O R
O O A O N N D I M T A L T S I G B
P A O L N A D F O L N Y O D K T I
S D C R T O B L U B E R H U T T E
W T A H E K O A O V E R R B I B O
B O V E E B P R W R L S F Y R B U
T U I T Q R O W U L T E O K W R T
U F T G P I K U E S I N R A O E U
O A Y B T I K E S H R E M X O P J
K T E T H T C F H R E G L E M C
S E B V F S E S W I R E A D P C
```

BRACES
SMILES
BAND
RETAINER
TEETH
DENTIST
ORTHODONTIST
IMPRESSION
BRACKET
APPLIANCE
OVERBITE
UNDERBITE
CAVITY
WAX
TOOTHBRUSH
BRUSH
FLOSS
MOLAR
WIRE
GUMS

Answers on page 42

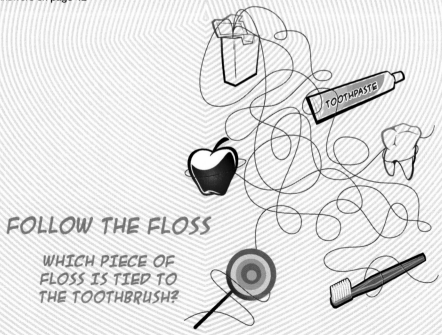

FOLLOW THE FLOSS

WHICH PIECE OF FLOSS IS TIED TO THE TOOTHBRUSH?

TOOTHPASTE

PICTURE CROSSWORD

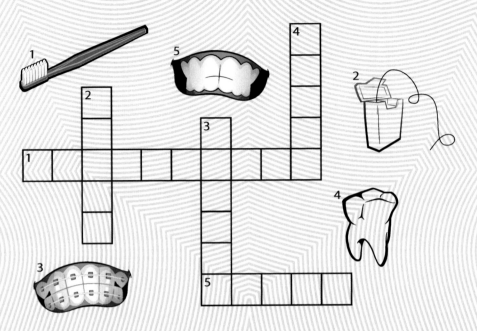

Answers on page 42

HOW MANY WORDS CAN YOU MAKE OUT OF THE WORD: TOOTHBRUSH?

EXAMPLE: BRUSH, TOOTH

TOOTH TRUTHS ANSWER KEY

1. B - The Orthodontist. Orthodontists can help you determine if you need braces to straighten your teeth and give you a glowing smile.

2. B - 32. Most kids have 20 baby teeth or primary teeth by age 3. Around ages 5 and 6, kids lose their baby teeth, and permanent teeth grow in their place. By age 14, most kids have 28 permanent teeth. Around 20, four wisdom grow in the back of the mouth, completing a total set of 32 teeth.

3. C - Every 6 months. Visiting the dentist every six months will help keep your teeth in tip top shape.

4. B - 2-3 minutes. Taking care of your teeth requires you to brush for 2-3 minutes to prevent cavities and tooth decay. Move your brush in small circles over the outsides of teeth, then brush the insides and tops of your teeth.

5. D - All of the above. Wearing braces can straighten any irregularities in the alignment of teeth. Misaligned teeth can lead to tooth decay, gum disease and can even cause headaches. Braces can also improve smiles.

6. A - Brush twice a day, floss and visit the dentist regularly. Brushing your teeth with a pea sized dab of fluoride toothpaste twice a day, flossing once a day and visiting the dentist every six months will help keep your teeth shiny and healthy.

7. C - Plaque. Taking care of your teeth will help remove plaque, a clear film that sticks to teeth. Plaque contains harmful bacteria that leads to cavities and tooth decay.

8. B - Malocclusion. Malocclusion means "bad bite" and is used by dentists and orthodontists to describe teeth that are crooked, crowded or improperly positioned.

THE TOOTH OF THE MATTER QUIZ ANSWER KEY

1. B - Acupuncture. Oral disease has been a problem for humans since early times. Cro-Magnon skulls from 25,000 years ago contain evidence of tooth decay.

2. C - Thread. Pierre Fauchard, a French surgeon, is also credited with being the "father of modern dentistry" and published a book that contained a chapter on teeth straightening.

3. A - Dental floss. Although prehistoric human teeth show some evidence of flossing, Levi Spear Parmly invented dental floss using silk thread. During World War II, Dr. Charles Bass developed nylon floss to replace silk floss.

4. C - Paul Revere. Along with silversmithing, Paul Revere practiced dentistry in colonial Boston. A surgeon dentist taught him how to clean teeth and to fix loose false teeth.

5. D - Barber. From the Middle Ages to the early 1700s, "barber surgeons" provided dental relief. In addition to cutting hair, these jacks-of-all-trades also extracted teeth and performed minor surgery.

6. B - Rouge. Vermilion rouge was made from a sulfur and mercury compound that caused inflamed gums and tooth loss.

7. C - Tooth powder. Ancient Romans used tooth powder that contained highly abrasive ingredients that made teeth appear shiny, but eroded the surface, exposing the pulp.

8. **A - George Washington.** Our first president insisted that the teeth of his six horses be cleaned and groomed daily to improve their appearance. Washington, on the other hand, had false teeth made of metal and carved ivory.

9. **D - All of the above.** Magical cures and bizarre attempts to relieve toothaches proliferated in the ancient past.

10. **B - Etruscans.** The Etruscans of central Italy, the fathers of much of what we know about Roman civilization, produced partial dentures of bridgework. Some dentures were removable for cleaning while others were permanently attached to the original surviving teeth.

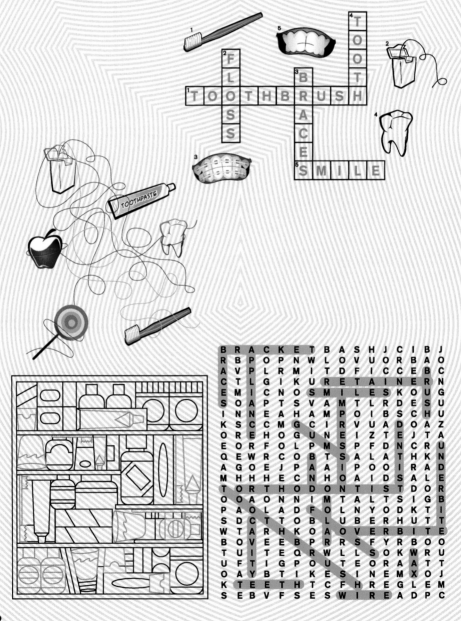